JUICING FOR LIVER HEALTH

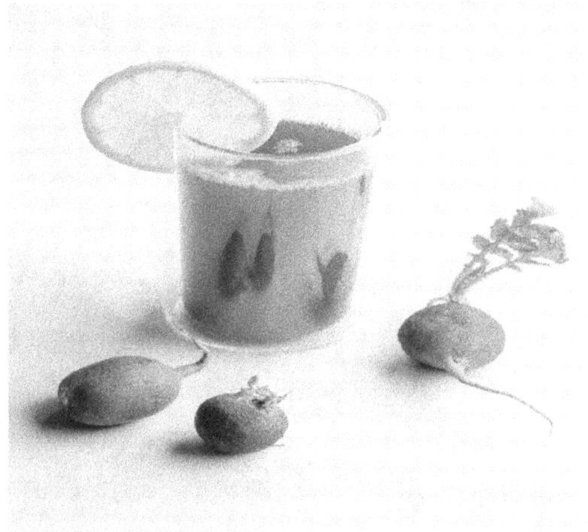

A comprehensive guide to cleansing, rejuvenating and detoxing your liver with Nutritious and delicious healthy juices and smoothies recipes

Shane Ramiro

Table of contents

Introduction

Nestled in the serene town of Harmony Grove, where the sun-dappled orchards sway with the rhythm of well-being, a quiet revolution is taking root. In this haven of health seekers, a humble juicery named "Harmony Greens" emerges as the heart of a community drawn together by a shared pursuit: juicing for liver health.

Enter Shane, a passionate wellness advocate and the visionary behind Harmony Greens. With an infectious enthusiasm, Shane guides patrons through the vibrant kaleidoscope of fruits and vegetables, each chosen for its unique contribution to liver vitality. The town, once captivated by convenience, now gathers at Harmony Greens, thirsty for the elixirs that promise not just flavor but a symphony of nourishment for their livers.

As patrons exchange stories of renewed energy and vitality, Shane becomes the storyteller-in-chief, weaving tales of the liver's resilience and its profound connection to overall health. The juicery's walls resonate with the murmur of cucumber-infused hydration and the hum of blenders crafting kale-packed concoctions—all designed to support the liver's intricate dance of detoxification.

Harmony Greens stands as a testament to the transformative power of juicing, where the pursuit of liver health intertwines with the community's fabric. The story unfolds with each sip, as the townsfolk embrace a holistic approach to well-being, savoring the sweet and savory blends that whisper promises of a

healthier, harmonious life.

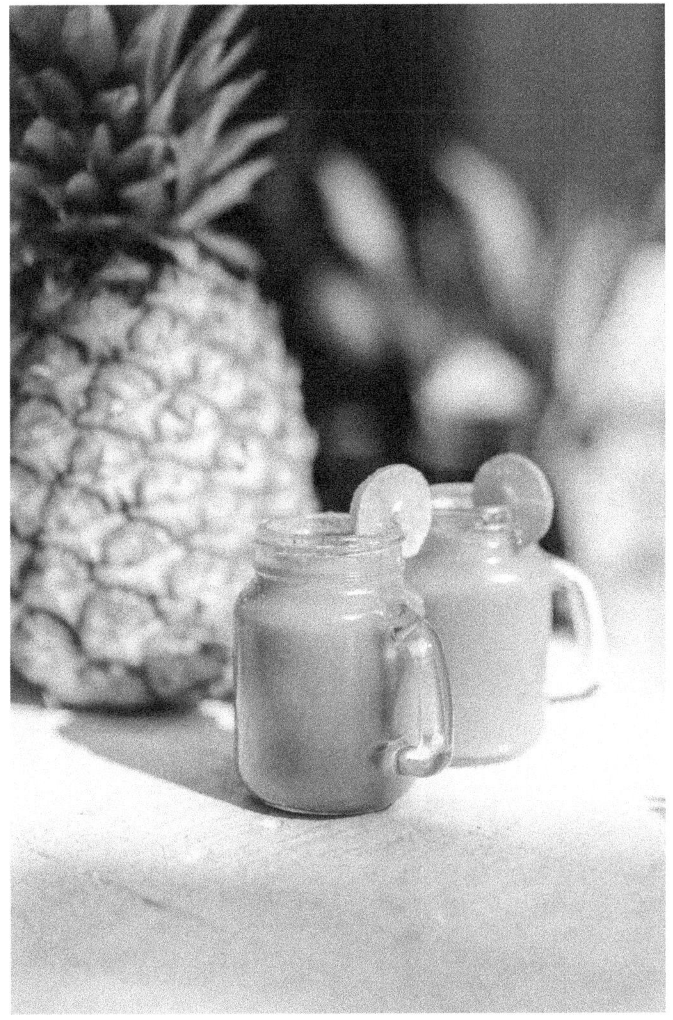

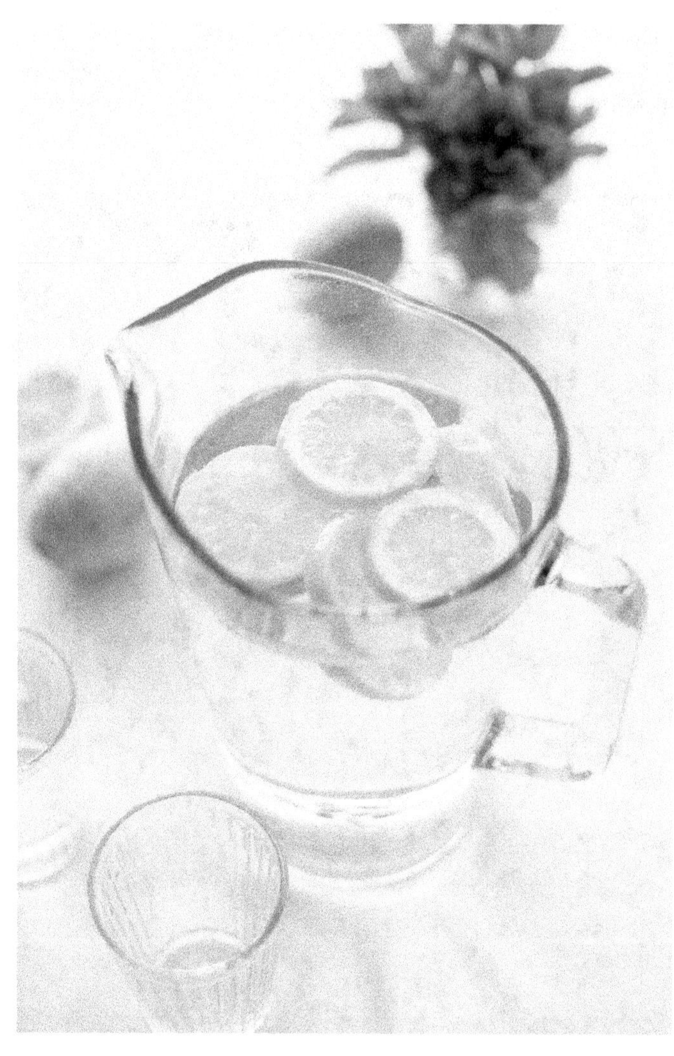

Chapter one

What is Liver

Located in the upper right side of the belly, the liver is an essential organ of the human body. It is the largest internal organ and plays a crucial role in numerous physiological processes, making it indispensable for overall health.

Key Aspects of the Liver:

1. Anatomy: The liver is a reddish-brown organ with a unique lobular structure. It consists of two main lobes, further divided into smaller lobules. Blood is supplied to the liver through the hepatic artery and portal vein.

2. Size: It is the largest internal organ in the body, weighing approximately 3 pounds in adults.

3. Location: Positioned just below the diaphragm, the liver is protected by the ribcage.

Functions:

The liver is a complex organ with multifaceted functions crucial for maintaining overall health. Its intricate workings involve a combination of metabolic, synthetic, and regulatory processes. Here's an overview of how the liver works:

1. Metabolism:
   - Carbohydrate Metabolism: The liver helps regulate blood glucose levels by storing excess glucose as glycogen or converting glycogen back to glucose when needed.

- Fat Metabolism: It plays a key role in lipid metabolism, synthesizing and breaking down fats. The liver also produces cholesterol and triglycerides.

2. Detoxification:

   - The liver filters and detoxifies blood by breaking down toxins, drugs, and metabolic byproducts. This detoxification process involves various enzymes and pathways, converting harmful substances into water-soluble compounds that can be excreted.

3. Protein Metabolism:

   - The liver synthesizes a variety of proteins, including blood-clotting factors, albumin (which helps maintain blood volume and pressure), and enzymes involved in digestion.

4. Bile Production:
   - Bile, a digestive fluid produced by the liver, facilitates the emulsification and absorption of lipids. Bile is stored in the gallbladder and discharged into the small intestine as required.

5. Storage:
   - The liver acts as a storage facility for essential nutrients and minerals, including vitamins (such as A, D, and B12), iron, and glycogen.

6. Blood Regulation:
   - The liver helps regulate blood composition by filtering and processing nutrients absorbed

from the digestive system. It adjusts nutrient levels to maintain balance and prevent harmful substances from entering the bloodstream.

7. Immune System Support:
   - Kupffer cells, specialized immune cells within the liver, help remove bacteria and other foreign particles from the blood, contributing to the body's defense against infections.

Common Liver Conditions:

1. Hepatitis: Inflammation of the liver, often caused by viral infections (hepatitis A, B, C).

2. Cirrhosis: Scarring of the liver tissue, usually a result of prolonged liver damage from conditions like alcoholism or chronic hepatitis.

3. Fatty Liver Disease: Accumulation of excess fat in the liver cells, often linked to obesity and metabolic syndrome.

4. Liver Cancer: The development of cancerous cells in the liver, which can be primary or metastatic.

Maintaining Liver Health:

A healthy lifestyle, including a balanced diet, regular exercise, limited alcohol consumption, and avoiding exposure to toxins, is crucial for maintaining optimal liver function.

Understanding the multifaceted role of the liver highlights its significance in sustaining overall health and emphasizes the importance of 15

adopting habits that support its well-being.

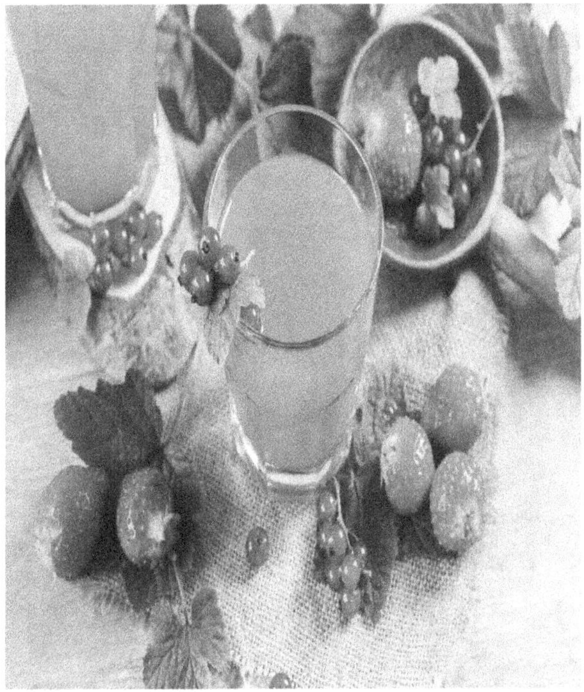

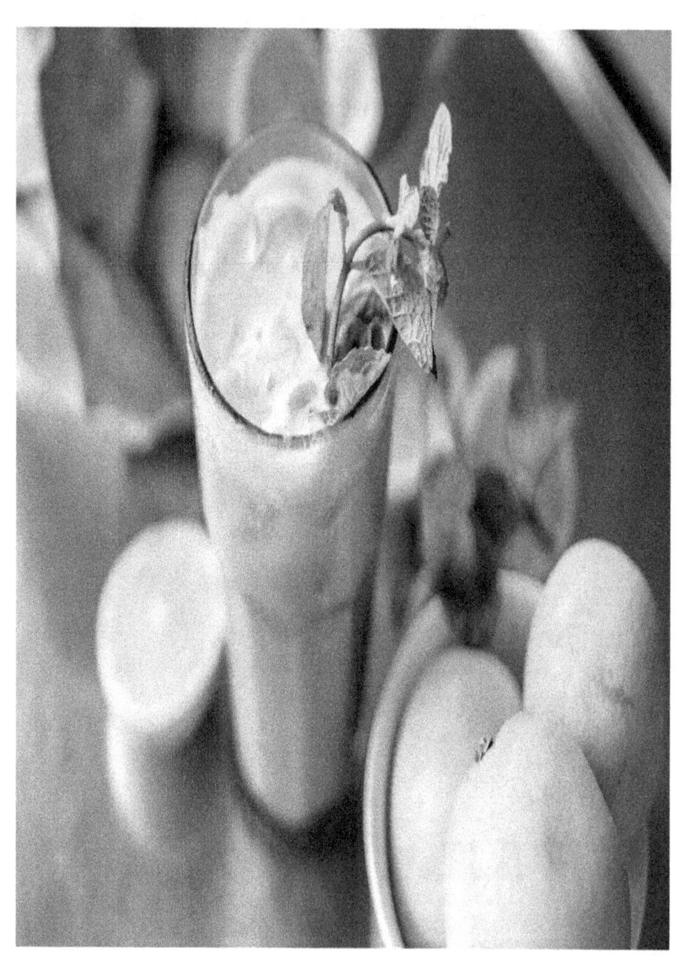

Chapter two

The Benefits of Juicing for the Liver

Juicing can offer several potential benefits for liver health when incorporated into a balanced and healthy lifestyle:

1. Nutrient Boost: Freshly juiced fruits and vegetables provide a concentrated source of vitamins, minerals, and antioxidants that support overall health and contribute to the liver's detoxification processes.

2. Hydration: Juicing can help maintain adequate hydration levels, which is essential for optimal liver function. Proper hydration supports the liver in flushing out toxins and aiding metabolic processes.

3. Liver Detoxification: Certain fruits and vegetables, such as beets, carrots, and leafy greens, contain compounds that may enhance the liver's natural detoxification mechanisms, promoting the elimination of harmful substances from the body.

4. Reduced Oxidative Stress: Antioxidants present in fruits and vegetables, such as vitamin C and E, help combat oxidative stress. By neutralizing free radicals, these antioxidants may protect liver cells from damage.

5. Anti-Inflammatory Properties: Some fruits and vegetables, like ginger and turmeric, possess anti-inflammatory properties. Chronic inflammation can contribute to liver damage, and

incorporating anti-inflammatory foods
may have a positive impact.

6. Improved Digestion: Juicing can provide
    a readily absorbable form of nutrients,
    aiding digestion and reducing the
    workload on the liver. The fiber in whole
    fruits and vegetables can also support a
    healthy digestive system.

7. Weight Management: Maintaining a
    healthy weight is crucial for liver health,
    as excess fat in the liver can lead to
    conditions like fatty liver disease. Juicing
    can be part of a balanced approach to
    weight management when combined
    with a nutritious diet and regular
    exercise.

It's important to note that while juicing can be a
beneficial component of a healthy lifestyle, it

should not replace whole fruits and vegetables in the diet. Whole foods provide essential fiber, which is often reduced in the juicing process. Additionally, consulting with a healthcare professional or a nutritionist before making significant dietary changes is advisable, especially for individuals with pre-existing health conditions.

Nutritional components of juicing

Juicing extracts and concentrates the nutritional components of fruits and vegetables, providing a potent and easily absorbable source of essential nutrients. The nutritional profile of freshly juiced produce includes:

1. Vitamins:

    - Vitamin C: Found in citrus fruits, strawberries, and kiwi, vitamin C

supports the immune system and
acts as an antioxidant, protecting
cells from damage.

- Vitamin A: Abundant in carrots,
sweet potatoes, and leafy greens,
vitamin A is crucial for vision, skin
health, and immune function.

2. Minerals:

- Potassium: Present in fruits like
bananas and oranges, potassium
helps regulate blood pressure
and supports proper muscle and
nerve function.

- Magnesium: Leafy greens, nuts,
and seeds contribute
magnesium, essential for muscle
and nerve function, as well as
bone health.

3. Antioxidants:

- Flavonoids: Abundant in berries, citrus fruits, and green tea, flavonoids have antioxidant properties that combat oxidative stress and inflammation.
- Carotenoids: Found in carrots, sweet potatoes, and kale, carotenoids are antioxidants that support skin health and may have anti-cancer properties.

4. Phytochemicals:

- Glucosinolates: Present in cruciferous vegetables like broccoli and kale, glucosinolates have potential anti-cancer effects and support liver detoxification.
- Polyphenols: Abundant in berries, apples, and green tea,

polyphenols possess antioxidant and anti-inflammatory properties.

5. Enzymes:
   - Digestive Enzymes: Juicing preserves enzymes naturally present in fruits and vegetables, aiding digestion and promoting nutrient absorption.

6. Fiber:
   - Soluble Fiber: While juicing removes much of the insoluble fiber, soluble fiber remains. This type of fiber, found in fruits like apples and pears, helps regulate blood sugar levels and lower cholesterol.

7. Hydration:
   - Juices contribute to overall hydration, supporting bodily

functions and promoting healthy skin.

It's important to note that while juicing offers a concentrated source of nutrients, whole fruits and vegetables should still be part of a balanced diet. The fiber in whole foods plays a crucial role in digestion and helps maintain a healthy gut.

Chapter three

Different types of juicing

There are various methods and types of juicing, each with its own characteristics and benefits. Here are some popular types of juicing:

1. Centrifugal Juicing:
    - How it works: Uses a fast-spinning blade to shred fruits and vegetables and extract juice.
    - Pros: Quick and efficient, suitable for most fruits and vegetables.
    - Cons: May generate some heat, potentially affecting nutrient content. Not ideal for leafy greens.

2. Masticating Juicing (Cold Press or Slow Juicing):

    o   How it works: Utilizes a slower rotating auger to crush and press fruits and vegetables, extracting juice.

    o   Pros: Preserves more nutrients due to lower heat production, extracts juice from leafy greens effectively.

    o   Cons: Slower compared to centrifugal juicing.

3. Twin Gear Juicing:

    o   How it works: Uses two interlocking gears to crush and press fruits and vegetables, extracting juice.

    o   Pros: Efficient extraction, retains more nutrients.

- Cons: Typically more expensive
     and bulkier than other juicers.

4. Hydraulic Press Juicing:
   - How it works: Crushes fruits and
     vegetables with thousands of
     pounds of pressure, extracting
     juice.
   - Pros: Yields high-quality juice
     with minimal heat, excellent
     nutrient retention.
   - Cons: Expensive and large, not
     as common for home use.

5. Blender Juicing (Whole Food Juicing):
   - How it works: Blends whole fruits
     and vegetables, producing a
     thicker beverage.
   - Pros: Retains fiber content,
     creating a smoother consistency.

- Cons: Can be less effective at extracting juice compared to traditional juicers.

6. Green Juicing:
   - Focus: Specifically emphasizes juicing with green vegetables, often including leafy greens like kale and spinach.
   - Benefits: High in chlorophyll, vitamins, and minerals, known for their potential detoxifying and health-promoting properties.

7. Fruit Juicing:
   - Focus: Emphasizes fruits, creating sweeter and often more palatable juices.
   - Benefits: Provides a natural sweetness and a variety of vitamins and antioxidants.

8. Detox Juicing:

  - Focus: Incorporates fruits and vegetables with detoxifying properties, such as beets, ginger, and lemon.
  - Benefits: Aims to support the body's natural detoxification processes.

When choosing a juicing method, consider your preferences, the types of produce you want to juice, and your desired outcome, whether it's nutrient density, taste, or specific health goals. Each method has its own merits, and the best one for you depends on your individual needs and lifestyle.

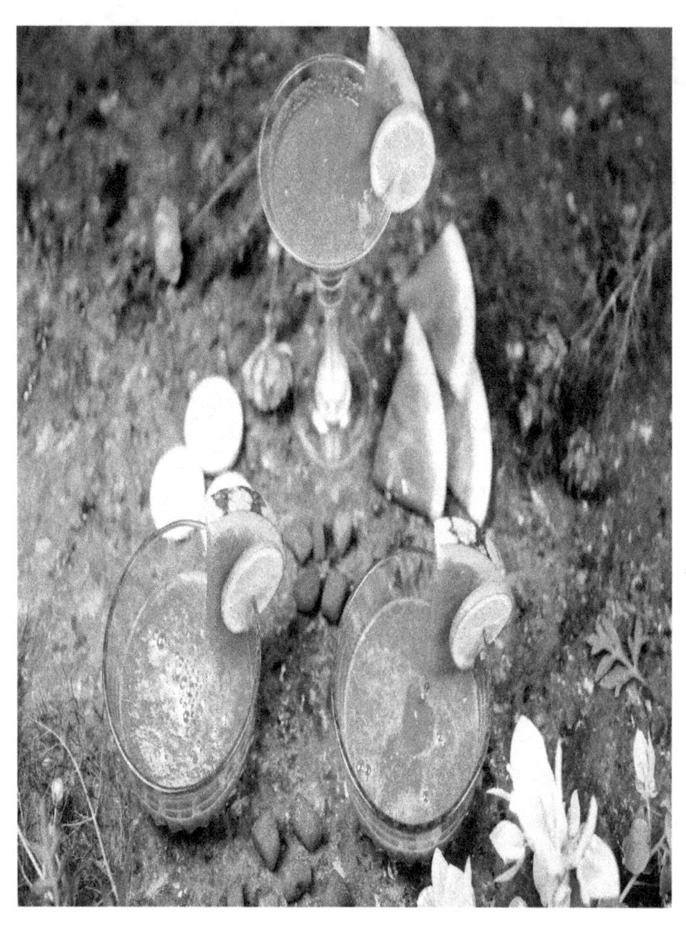

Chapter four

BEST PRACTICES FOR JUICING

How To Choose The Right Juicer

Choosing the right juicing method involves considering your preferences, lifestyle, and health goals. Here are factors to keep in mind when selecting a juicing approach:

1. Type of Juicer:
   - Centrifugal Juicers: Fast and efficient, suitable for most fruits and vegetables. Ideal for those seeking quick and convenient juicing.
   - Masticating Juicers (Cold Press): Slower, preserving more nutrients and extracting juice from leafy

greens. Suitable for those willing to spend a bit more time on juicing for higher nutritional value.

2. Budget:

    o   Consider the cost of the juicer and the ongoing expense of purchasing fresh produce. Centrifugal juicers are generally more affordable, while masticating and twin gear juicers tend to be pricier.

3. Nutrient Retention:

    o   If retaining maximum nutrients is a priority, masticating, twin gear, and hydraulic press juicers are known for their ability to minimize heat during the juicing process, preserving more enzymes and nutrients.

4. Ease of Cleaning:

    o   Since centrifugal juicers have a
        simpler construction, they are
        often easier to clean. Consider
        the cleaning process and how
        much time you are willing to
        dedicate to maintenance.

5. Juice Texture:

    o   If you prefer a smoother juice
        consistency with minimal pulp,
        centrifugal juicers are suitable. If
        you enjoy a thicker juice with
        more fiber, consider using a
        blender or masticating juicer.

6. Space Considerations:

    o   Some juicers are bulkier than
        others. If kitchen space is limited,
        a compact centrifugal juicer or a
        blender might be more practical.

7. Juicing Goals:

    o   Consider your specific health
        goals. If detoxification is a priority,
        you might opt for detox-focused
        juicing with ingredients like beets
        and ginger. For nutrient-dense
        green juices, a masticating juicer
        is often recommended.

8. Frequency of Use:

    o   If you plan to juice regularly,
        invest in a durable and reliable
        juicer. Consider the warranty and
        reviews to ensure the longevity of
        the appliance.

9. Versatility:

    o   Some juicers are versatile and
        can handle a variety of produce,
        while others may be more
        specialized. Choose based on

the types of fruits and vegetables you enjoy juicing.

10. Noise Level:

- Centrifugal juicers tend to be noisier than masticating juicers. If noise is a concern, consider a quieter option, especially if you plan to juice early in the morning or late at night.

Ultimately, the right juicing method is a personal choice that aligns with your lifestyle, preferences, and health objectives. It's beneficial to research and perhaps even try different juicing methods to discover which one best suits your needs.

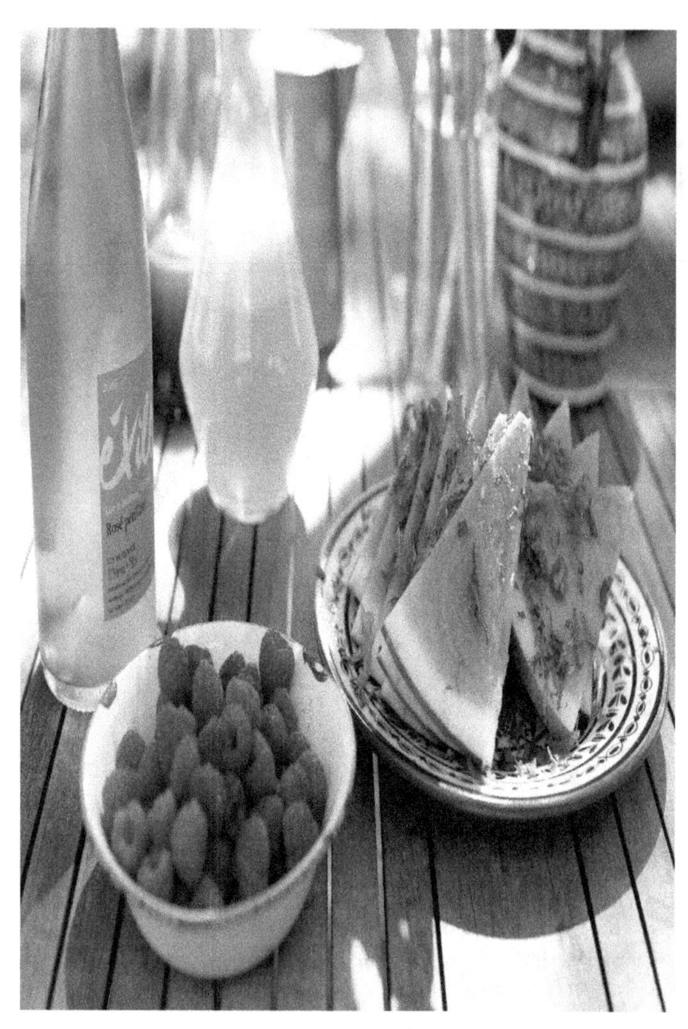

Chapter five

How to Choose the Right Ingredients

When choosing ingredients for juicing to support liver health, focus on incorporating a variety of fruits, vegetables, and herbs known for their liver-boosting properties. Here's a guide on selecting the right ingredients:

1. Leafy Greens:
    - Examples: Kale, spinach, collard greens, and Swiss chard.
    - Benefits: Rich in chlorophyll and antioxidants, leafy greens support liver detoxification.
2. Cruciferous Vegetables:

- Examples: Broccoli, Brussels sprouts, cauliflower, and cabbage.
- Benefits: Contain glucosinolates, which aid in liver detoxification and promote overall liver health.

3. Citrus Fruits:

- Examples: Lemons, limes, oranges, and grapefruits.
- Benefits: High in vitamin C and antioxidants, citrus fruits support the immune system and liver function.

4. Beets:

- Benefits: Contains betaine, which may help protect the liver from oxidative stress, and supports the liver's natural detoxification processes.

5. Carrots:

   - Benefits: Rich in beta-carotene and antioxidants, carrots promote liver health and support overall well-being.

6. Ginger:

   - Benefits: Possesses anti-inflammatory and antioxidant properties, supporting liver function and digestion.

7. Turmeric:

   - Benefits: Contains curcumin, known for its anti-inflammatory and antioxidant effects, which may benefit liver health.

8. Apples:

   - Benefits: High in soluble fiber, apples aid digestion and help

regulate blood sugar levels,
benefiting the liver.

9. Celery:

   ○ Benefits: Has anti-inflammatory
   properties and is rich in
   antioxidants, contributing to liver
   health.

10. Dandelion Greens:

   ○ Benefits: Known for their potential
   to support liver detoxification and
   promote bile production.

11. Mint:

   ○ Benefits: Adds a refreshing flavor
   and may help soothe the
   digestive system.

12. Cucumber:

   ○ Benefits: Hydrating and low in
   calories, cucumber can be a

refreshing addition to liver-supportive juices.

When combining ingredients, aim for a balance of flavors and textures to create a palatable juice. Additionally, consider including a variety of colors, as different colors often indicate diverse nutrient profiles.

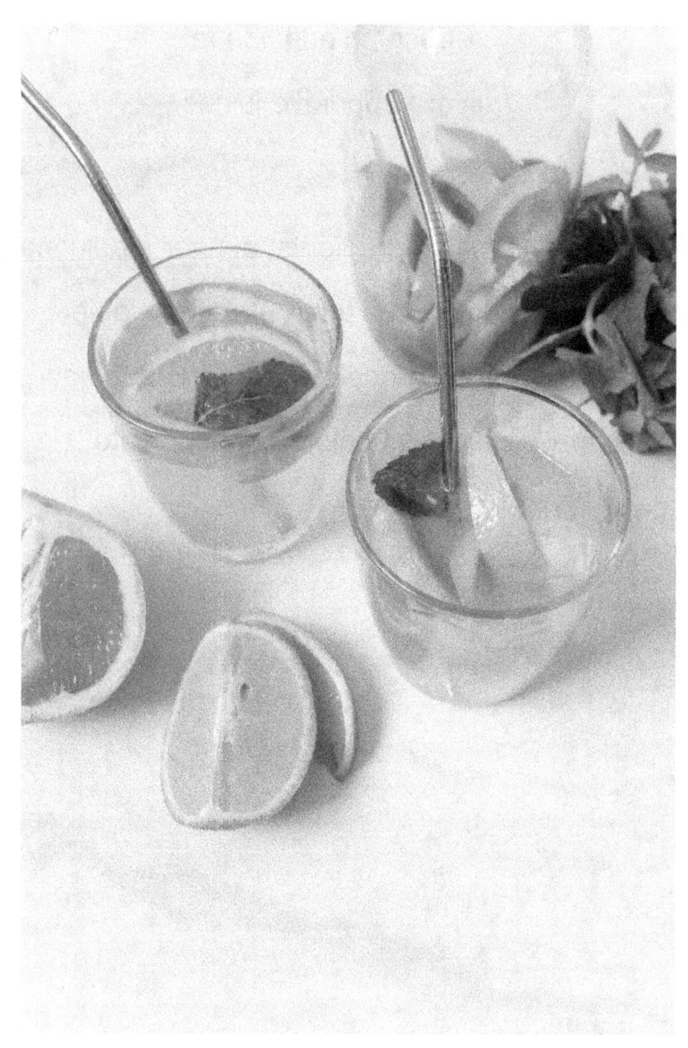

Chapter six

Good safety consideration

Maintaining food safety during juicing is crucial to prevent contamination and ensure the health benefits of the juice. Here are some key considerations for ensuring food safety in juicing for liver health:

1. Wash Produce Thoroughly:
    - Rinse fruits and vegetables under cold running water before juicing to remove dirt, bacteria, and pesticides. Use a brush for items with thicker skins, like carrots or cucumbers.
2. Choose Fresh, High-Quality Produce:
    - Choose premium, fresh fruit to reduce the chance of infection.

Avoid using fruits or vegetables that show signs of spoilage or damage.

3. Clean Cutting Boards and Utensils:

    - Wash cutting boards, knives, and other utensils with hot soapy water before and after preparing ingredients for juicing. This helps prevent cross-contamination.

4. Use Clean Hands:

    - Wash your hands thoroughly with soap and water before handling produce or operating the juicer to avoid introducing harmful bacteria.

5. Keep Juicing Equipment Clean:

    - Regularly clean and sanitize all parts of your juicer according to the manufacturer's instructions.

Pay extra attention to areas where juice or pulp may accumulate.

6. Handle Raw Eggs and Dairy Products Safely:
   - If your juicing recipe includes raw eggs or dairy, ensure they are pasteurized to reduce the risk of foodborne illnesses. Use reputable sources for these products.

7. Refrigerate Perishable Ingredients:
   - If you prepare juice in advance or store leftover ingredients, refrigerate them promptly to inhibit the growth of harmful bacteria. Consume refrigerated juice within a recommended timeframe.

8. Avoid Cross-Contamination:

   o Keep raw meat, poultry, and
     seafood separate from fruits and
     vegetables. Use different cutting
     boards and utensils for raw
     animal products to avoid
     cross-contamination.

9. Be Mindful of Allergens:

   o If you or others consuming the
     juice have allergies, be vigilant
     about potential allergens present
     in the ingredients. Clearly label
     any allergenic components.

10. Be Aware of Expiry Dates:

   o Check the expiration dates on
     packaged items like nut milks or
     other ingredients. Using expired
     products may pose health risks.

11. Consume Freshly Juiced Beverages
Promptly:

- For the best flavor and nutritional
  value, consume freshly juiced
  beverages soon after
  preparation. Use airtight
  containers and quickly chill if
  storing.

By following these food safety considerations,
you can enjoy the health benefits of juicing
while minimizing the risk of foodborne
illnesses. Always prioritize cleanliness, fresh
ingredients, and proper storage to create safe
and nutritious liver-supportive juices.

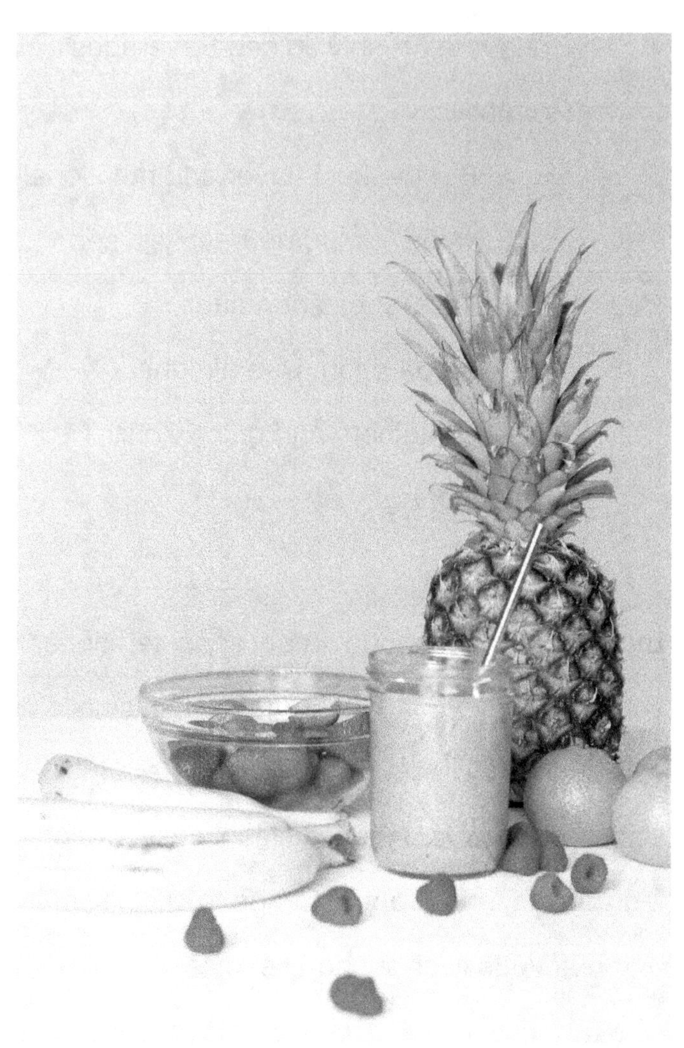

Chapter seven

How To Store Your Juice

Storing freshly made juice properly is essential to maintain its freshness, flavor, and nutritional value. Here are some guidelines on how to store your juice:

1. Refrigerate Promptly:
   - After juicing, transfer the juice to a clean, airtight container and refrigerate it immediately. Exposure to air and light can lead to nutrient loss and oxidation, so sealing the container tightly is crucial.
2. Use Glass Containers:
   - Glass containers are preferable over plastic for storing juice

because they don't absorb odors
or leach chemicals into the juice.
Choose containers with a
tight-sealing lid to minimize
exposure to air.

3. Fill Containers to the Top:

    o   To minimize air exposure, fill your
        storage container to the brim,
        leaving as little space as possible
        at the top. This helps reduce
        oxidation.

4. Store in a Dark, Cool Place:

    o   If your juice is in a transparent
        container, store it in a dark place,
        like the back of the refrigerator.
        Light can degrade certain
        nutrients and affect the quality of
        the juice.

5. Consume Within 24-48 Hours:

- Freshly made juice is most nutritious when consumed shortly after preparation. While some juices may stay fresh for up to 72 hours, it's generally best to consume them within the first 24-48 hours to maximize their benefits.

6. Freeze for Extended Storage:

   - If you want to store juice for a more extended period, consider freezing it. Use airtight, freezer-safe containers, leaving some space for expansion. Thaw frozen juice in the refrigerator before consuming.

7. Shake Before Drinking:

   - Natural separation can occur over time, especially if the juice

contains different types of
ingredients. Shake or stir the
juice well before drinking to remix
any settled particles.

8. Choose Juicing Ingredients Wisely:

    o Some ingredients oxidize more
       quickly than others. Citrus fruits,
       for example, are prone to
       oxidation. Consider this when
       planning your juice and try to
       consume those types of juices
       more promptly.

9. Avoid Metal Containers:

    o Avoid using metal containers for
       storing juice, as metals can react
       with certain compounds in the
       juice and alter the taste.

10. Monitor Signs of Spoilage:

- Look for any variations in taste, smell, or color. If the juice develops an off-putting smell, taste, or appearance, it's best to discard it.

By following these storage guidelines, you can prolong the freshness and nutritional quality of your freshly made juice. Remember that while juicing is a great way to enjoy the benefits of fruits and vegetables, consuming whole fruits and vegetables is also important for a well-rounded diet.

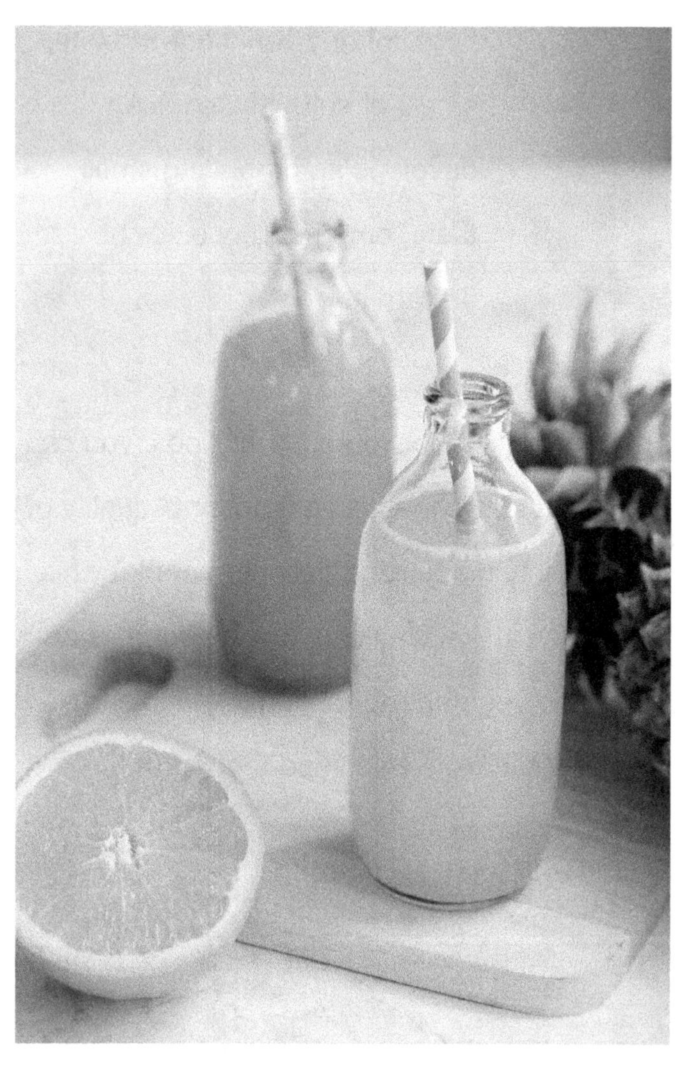

Chapter eight

Liver Detox Recipes

Liver detox recipes are designed to incorporate ingredients that are believed to support the liver's natural detoxification processes. While the concept of "detoxing" should be approached with caution, as the liver is a self-regulating organ, consuming nutrient-dense foods can contribute to overall health. Here's a comprehensive guide to liver detox recipes:

1. Green Detox Juice:

- Ingredients:
    - 1 cucumber, peeled and sliced
    - 2 celery stalks

- Handful of fresh parsley and cilantro
    - 1 green apple, cored and sliced
    - 1/2 lemon, peeled
    - 1-inch piece of fresh ginger
    - 1 cup of spinach or kale
- Instructions:
    - Juice all ingredients and stir well. Drink immediately for maximum freshness.

2. Beet and Carrot Liver Cleanse:

- Ingredients:
    - 1 medium-sized beet, peeled and sliced
    - 2 large carrots, peeled and sliced
    - 1 apple, cored and sliced
    - 1/2 lemon, peeled

- - 1-inch piece of fresh ginger

- Instructions:

    - Juice all ingredients, mix well, and enjoy the vibrant liver-supporting blend.

3. Turmeric Elixir:

- Ingredients:

    - 1 tablespoon fresh turmeric root, grated (or 1 teaspoon turmeric powder)
    - 1 tablespoon fresh ginger, grated
    - 1/2 lemon, juiced
    - Dash of black pepper (to enhance turmeric absorption)
    - 1 teaspoon honey (optional)
    - 2 cups warm water

- Instructions:

- Mix all ingredients in warm water. Stir well and sip slowly.

4. Citrus Bliss Infusion:

- Ingredients:
  - 1 orange, peeled and segmented
  - 1 grapefruit, peeled and segmented
  - 1 lemon, peeled and sliced
  - 1 lime, peeled and sliced
  - 1-2 sprigs of fresh mint
- Instructions:
  - Combine all citrus fruits and mint in a pitcher of water.Store in the refrigerator for a few hours or overnight to allow it to infuse. Enjoy a refreshing, hydrating drink.

5. Dandelion Greens Detox Smoothie:

- Ingredients:
    - 1 cup dandelion greens
    - 1/2 cucumber
    - 1/2 cup pineapple chunks
    - 1 green apple, cored and sliced
    - 1 tablespoon chia seeds
    - Coconut water or water for blending
- Instructions:
    - Blend all ingredients until smooth. Add more liquid if needed. Consume as a nutrient-packed smoothie.

Additional Tips:

- Stay Hydrated: Water is crucial for the detoxification process. Water is your best beverage throughout the day.
- Limit Processed Foods: Reduce intake of processed foods, added sugars, and alcohol during a detox period.
- Listen to Your Body: Pay attention to how your body responds and adjust ingredients based on personal preferences and sensitivities.

It's important to note that individual reactions to detox recipes can vary. If you have existing health concerns or are on medication, consult with a healthcare professional before embarking on a detox program. Incorporating these liver-friendly recipes as part of a balanced and varied diet is a sustainable approach to supporting overall health.

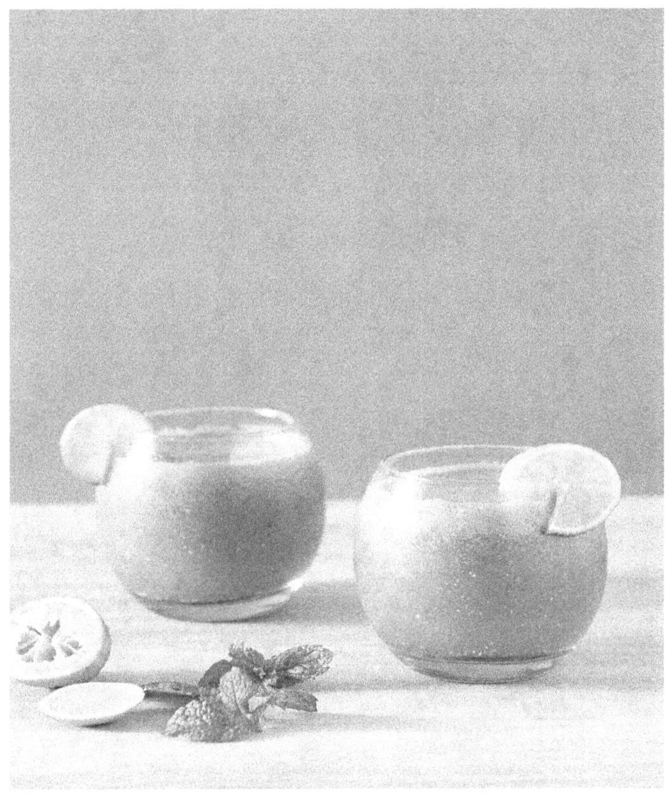

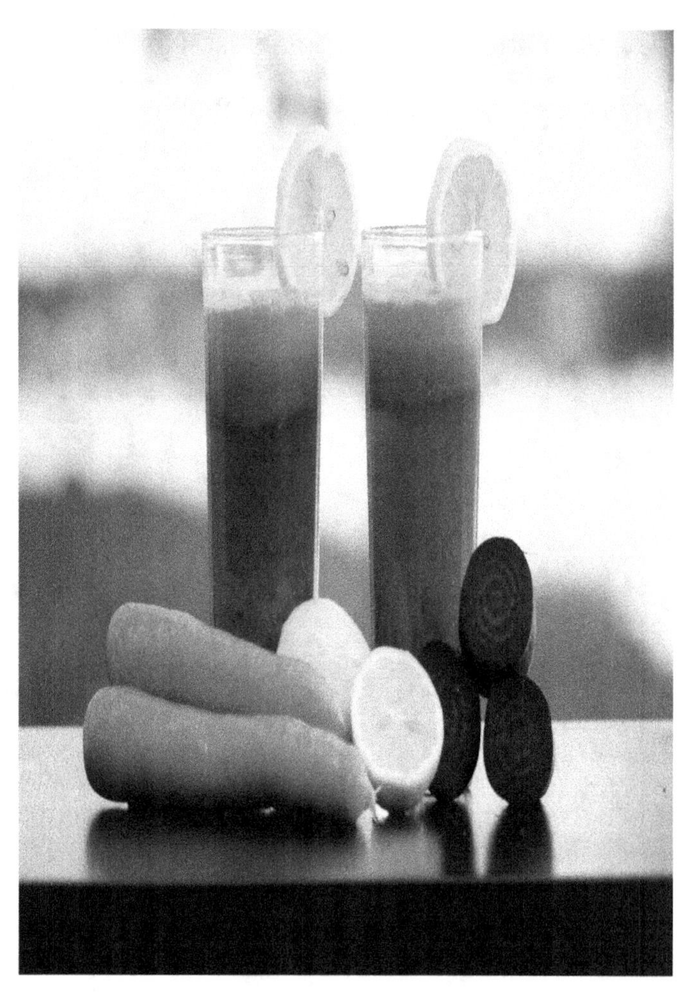

Chapter nine

Liver Repair Recipes

While the liver is a self-healing organ, incorporating foods that are supportive of liver health can aid in its repair and regeneration. Here's a comprehensive guide to liver repair recipes:

1. Liver-Boosting Green Smoothie:

- Ingredients:
    - 1 cup kale or spinach
    - 1/2 cucumber
    - 1 green apple, cored and sliced
    - 1/2 lemon, peeled
    - 1-inch piece of fresh ginger
    - 1 tablespoon chia seeds
    - 1 cup coconut water or water

- Instructions:

  - Blend all ingredients until smooth. This smoothie is rich in antioxidants and nutrients that support liver function.

2. Beet and Berry Liver Cleanse Juice:

- Ingredients:

  - 1 medium-sized beet, peeled and sliced
  - 1 cup mixed berries (blueberries, strawberries, raspberries)
  - 1/2 lemon, peeled
  - 1 tablespoon fresh mint leaves
  - 1 tablespoon flaxseeds
  - 1 cup water or coconut water
- Instructions:

- Juice the beet, berries, lemon, and mint. Blend the juice with flaxseeds and water. Antioxidants and anti-inflammatory qualities abound in this cuisine.

3. Turmeric-Ginger Liver Tonic:

- Ingredients:
  - One tablespoon of freshly grated turmeric (or one teaspoon of powdered turmeric)
  - 1 tablespoon fresh ginger, grated
  - 1 lemon, juiced
  - 1 teaspoon honey (optional)
  - 2 cups warm water
- Instructions:
  - Mix turmeric, ginger, lemon juice, and honey in warm water. Sip this

tonic for its anti-inflammatory and detoxifying effects.

4. Garlic and Lemon Detox Drink:

- Ingredients:
    - 1 garlic clove, minced
    - 1 lemon, juiced
    - 1 teaspoon raw honey
    - 1 cup warm water
- Instructions:
    - Mix minced garlic, lemon juice, and honey in warm water. Consume this drink in the morning on an empty stomach for potential liver-supportive benefits.

5. Cruciferous Veggie Stir-Fry:

- Ingredients:

  - Broccoli florets

  - Cauliflower florets

  - Brussels sprouts, halved

  - Kale, chopped

  - Garlic, minced

  - Olive oil

- Instructions:

  - Sauté garlic in olive oil, add the cruciferous vegetables, and stir-fry until tender. Cruciferous veggies contain compounds that may support liver health.

6. Baked Salmon with Turmeric:

- Ingredients:

  - Salmon fillets

  - 1 tablespoon olive oil

- 1 teaspoon turmeric powder

  - Lemon wedges

- Instructions:

  - Rub salmon fillets with olive oil
    and turmeric. Bake until cooked.
    Salmon provides omega-3 fatty
    acids, supporting overall health,
    including the liver.

Additional Tips:

- Hydration: Water is crucial for the
  detoxification process, so stay
  well-hydrated throughout the day.
- Fiber-Rich Foods: Include foods high in
  fiber, such as whole grains, fruits, and
  vegetables, to support digestion and
  liver function.

- Limit Processed Foods: Reduce intake of processed foods, added sugars, and alcohol during a liver repair period.

- Consult a Professional: If you have liver conditions or concerns, consult with a healthcare professional before making significant dietary changes.

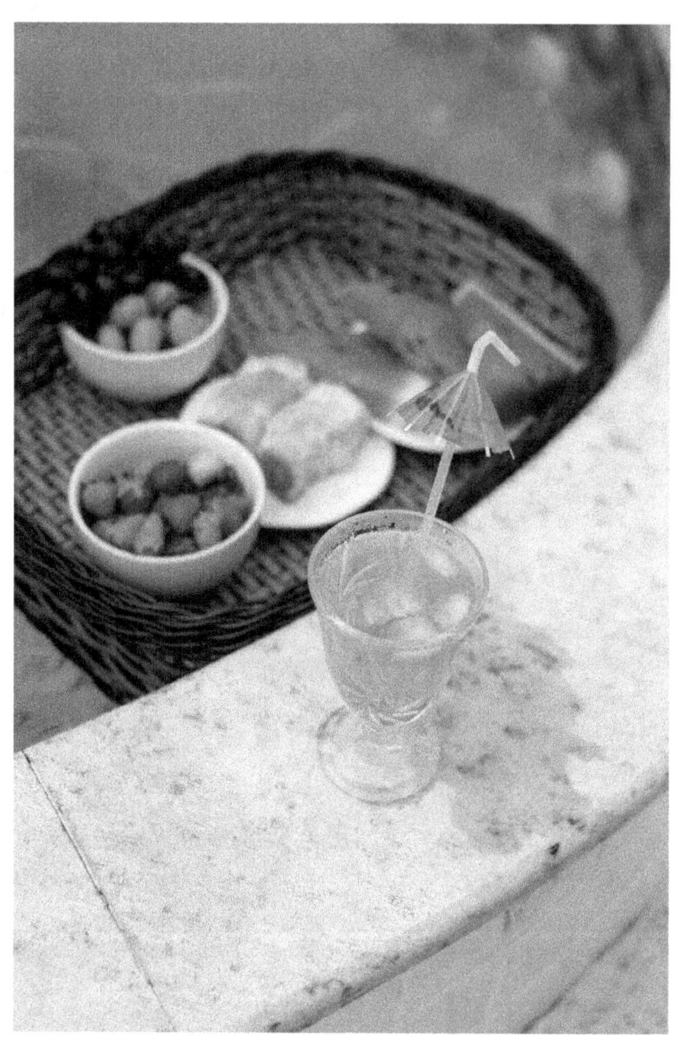

Chapter ten

Smoothie Recipes

Smoothies are versatile, delicious, and offer a convenient way to pack essential nutrients into your diet. Whether you're looking for a refreshing breakfast option, a post-workout snack, or a wholesome meal replacement, smoothies can be tailored to meet various tastes and nutritional needs. Here's an extensive guide to smoothie recipes with different themes and flavors:

**1. Green Goddess Smoothie:

- Ingredients:
    - 1 cup spinach or kale
    - 1/2 cucumber
    - 1 green apple, cored and sliced

- 1/2 lemon, peeled
    - 1-inch piece of fresh ginger
    - 1 tablespoon chia seeds
    - 1 cup coconut water or water
- Instructions:
    - Blend all ingredients until smooth. This nutrient-packed green smoothie is rich in antioxidants and fiber.

**2. Tropical Paradise Smoothie:

- Ingredients:
    - 1 cup pineapple chunks
    - 1/2 banana
    - 1/2 mango, peeled and diced
    - 1/2 cup coconut milk
    - 1/2 cup Greek yogurt
    - Ice cubes (optional)

- Instructions:

    - Blend all ingredients until smooth. Enjoy a taste of the tropics with this delicious and creamy smoothie.

**3. Berry Bliss Smoothie:

- Ingredients:

    - 1 cup mixed berries (strawberries, blueberries, raspberries)
    - 1/2 cup plain yogurt
    - 1/2 cup almond milk
    - 1 tablespoon honey
    - 1 tablespoon flaxseeds
    - Ice cubes (optional)
- Instructions:

- Blend all ingredients until smooth.
    This antioxidant-rich smoothie is
    both delicious and nutritious.

**4. Chocolate Peanut Butter Protein
Smoothie:

- Ingredients:
    - 1 banana
    - 2 tablespoons peanut butter
    - 1 scoop chocolate protein powder
    - 1 cup almond milk
    - Ice cubes (optional)
- Instructions:
    - Blend all ingredients until smooth.
      This high-protein smoothie is
      ideal for recuperating after a
      workout.

**5. Detoxifying Beet and Berry Smoothie:

- Ingredients:

    - 1 medium-sized beet, peeled and sliced

    - 1 cup mixed berries (blueberries, strawberries)

    - 1/2 cucumber

    - 1/2 lemon, peeled

    - 1 tablespoon chia seeds

    - 1 cup coconut water or water

- Instructions:

    - Blend all ingredients until smooth. This vibrant smoothie is loaded with antioxidants and may support detoxification.

**6. Minty Matcha Smoothie:

- Ingredients:

  - 1 teaspoon matcha powder

  - Handful of fresh mint leaves

  - 1/2 banana

  - 1/2 cup pineapple chunks

  - 1/2 cup Greek yogurt

  - 1 cup almond milk

  - Ice cubes (optional)

- Instructions:

  - Blend all ingredients until smooth. This energizing smoothie combines the goodness of matcha and the freshness of mint.

**7. Creamy Avocado Spinach Smoothie:

- Ingredients:

  - 1/2 avocado

- o   1 cup spinach
- o   1/2 banana
- o   1/2 cup Greek yogurt
- o   1 tablespoon chia seeds
- o   1 cup coconut water or water
- Instructions:
  - o   Blend all ingredients until smooth. This smoothie has a creamy texture and is high in good fats.

**8. Golden Turmeric Smoothie:

- Ingredients:
  - o   One tsp powdered turmeric (or freshly grated turmeric)
  - o   1/2 banana
  - o   1/2 cup mango chunks
  - o   1/2 cup plain yogurt
  - o   1 tablespoon honey

- 1 cup almond milk
- Instructions:
    - Blend all ingredients until smooth. This smoothie features the anti-inflammatory benefits of turmeric.

**9. Citrus Sunrise Smoothie:

- Ingredients:
    - 1 orange, peeled and segmented
    - 1/2 grapefruit, peeled and segmented
    - 1/2 cup Greek yogurt
    - 1 tablespoon honey
    - Ice cubes (optional)
- Instructions:

- ○ Blend all ingredients until smooth. This citrusy smoothie provides a burst of vitamin C.

**10. Pineapple Ginger Turmeric Smoothie:

- Ingredients:
    - ○ 1 cup pineapple chunks
    - ○ 1-inch piece of fresh ginger
    - ○ 1 teaspoon turmeric powder
    - ○ 1/2 cup coconut milk
    - ○ 1/2 cup plain yogurt
    - ○ Ice cubes (optional)
- Instructions:
    - ○ Blend all ingredients until smooth. This immune-boosting smoothie combines the flavors of pineapple, ginger, and turmeric.

Tips for Perfect Smoothies:

- Use Frozen Fruits: Frozen fruits add thickness and make the smoothie chilled without diluting the flavor.

- Include Protein: Add sources of protein like yogurt, nut butter, or protein powder for a satisfying and filling smoothie.

- Experiment with Liquids: Try different liquids like almond milk, coconut water, or green tea for varied flavors.

Conclusion

In conclusion, juicing for liver health offers a flavorful and nutritious approach to supporting the body's natural detoxification processes. Incorporating a variety of fruits, vegetables, and herbs in carefully crafted recipes can provide essential vitamins, minerals, antioxidants, and phytochemicals that contribute to overall liver well-being.

The liver, a vital organ with remarkable regenerative abilities, benefits from the inclusion of liver-friendly ingredients known for their potential detoxifying and anti-inflammatory properties. Green juices, rich in chlorophyll from leafy greens, and vibrant blends featuring beets, citrus fruits, and turmeric, are among the many options that can offer a nutritional boost while appealing to diverse tastes.

While the concept of "detoxing" should be approached with caution, as the liver naturally detoxifies the body, the mindful incorporation of nutrient-dense juices can be part of a balanced and health-conscious lifestyle. These juices, when combined with proper hydration, a fiber-rich diet, and a reduction in processed foods, contribute to holistic liver support.

It's essential to recognize that individual responses to dietary changes can vary, and consulting with a healthcare professional is advisable, especially for those with pre-existing health conditions. Moreover, focusing on long-term habits rather than short-term fixes ensures a sustainable approach to liver health.

In the realm of juicing, creativity knows no bounds. From green goddess smoothies to vibrant detoxifying elixirs, the world of juicing offers an array of flavors and nutritional benefits. Whether you're sipping on a refreshing green concoction or indulging in a berry-packed antioxidant blend, each sip brings you one step closer to a nourished and thriving liver.

So, let the colors of nature fill your glass, and embrace the wholesome goodness of juicing for liver health as a delightful journey toward overall well-being.

www.ingramcontent.com/pod-product-compliance
Lightning Source LLC
Chambersburg PA
CBHW061004260726

48661CB00005B/2054